STATEMENT

1994

on

Psychiatric-Mental Health Clinical Nursing Practice

and

STANDARDS

of

Psychiatric-Mental Health Clinical Nursing Practice

American Nurses Association
Council on Psychiatric and Mental Health Nursing

American Psychiatric Nurses Association

Association of Child and Adolescent Psychiatric Nurses

Society for Education and Research in Psychiatric-Mental
Health Nursing

This document is a collaborative effort of the members of the **Coalition of Psychiatric Nursing Organizations,** under the leadership of the Executive Committee of the American Nurses Association's (ANA) Council on Psychiatric and Mental Health Nursing. The Council gratefully acknowledges all the valuable assistance given by various individuals and groups across the country who have contributed comments and recommendations throughout the revision process.

Task Force to Revise Statement on Psychiatric-Mental Health Nursing Practice and Standards of Psychiatric-Mental Health Clinical Nursing Practice
Carolyn V. Billings, M.S.N., R.N.,C.S., *Chairperson*
ANA Council on Psychiatric and Mental Health Nursing
Jean Blackburn, M.S.N., R.N., C.S.
ANA Council on Psychiatric and Mental Health Nursing
Mickie Crimone, M.S., R.N., C.S.
Society for Education and Research in Psychiatric-Mental Health Nursing
Carol Dashiff, Ph.D., R.N., C.S.
Association for Child and Adolescent Psychiatric Nurses
Anita O'Toole, Ph.D., R.N., C.S., F.A.A.N.
ANA Council on Psychiatric and Mental Health Nursing
Kathleen Scharer, M.S., R.N., C.S., F.A.A.N.
ANA Committee on Nursing Practice Standards and Guidelines
Carole A. Shea, Ph.D., R.N., C.S.
American Psychiatric Nurses Association

Contributors
Margery Chisholm, Ed.D., R.N., C.S.
Sandra J. Fitzgerald, B.S.N., R.N., C.

Executive Committee, ANA Council on Psychiatric and Mental Health Nursing
Carolyn V. Billings, M.S.N., R.N., C.S., *Chairperson*
Christina Sieloff, M.S.N., R.N., C.N.A. *Chair-elect*
Jean Blackburn, M.S.N., R.N., C.S.
Beverly Farnsworth, Ph.D., R.N., C.S.
Judith Haber, Ph.D., R.N., C.S., F.A.A.N.
H. Marie McGrath, Ph.D., R.N.

Staff: ANA Department of Practice, Economics, and Policy
Sarah Stanley, M.S., R.N., C.N.A., C.S., Senior Policy Analyst
Valarie Carty, *Administrative Assistant*

ISBN 1-55810-098-9

Published by
American Nurses Publishing
600 Maryland Avenue, SW
Suite 100 West
Washington, DC 20024–2571

CONTENTS

PREFACE

The Executive Committee of the American Nurses Association's (ANA) Council on Psychiatric and Mental Health Nursing convened the 1992 Task Force to Revise the Statement and Standards of Psychiatric-Mental Health Nursing Practice. This revision, coordinated by the ANA council, is the joint effort of the members of the Coalition of Psychiatric Nursing Organizations (COPNO). COPNO includes the ANA Council on Psychiatric and Mental Health Nursing, the American Psychiatric Nurses Association, the Association of Child and Adolescent Psychiatric Nurses, and the Society for Education and Research in Psychiatric-Mental Health Nursing. Each of these organizations focuses on different aspects of the specialty and many nurses are members of more than one.

INTRODUCTION

In 1967, ANA's Division of Psychiatric and Mental Health Nursing Practice published the *Statement on Psychiatric Nursing Practice* (ANA 1967). ANA published a revision of this statement in 1976 (ANA 1976). Current trends and developments in the practice of nursing, in concert with issues and advances in the broader field of mental health care delivery, have highlighted the need to review and interpret the responsibilities of nurses within the specialty, particularly in regard to clinical practice. As a result, this revision focuses entirely on the clinical aspects of psychiatric-mental health nursing practice.

In the belief that scope of practice is inextricably linked to practice standards, this book also incorporates a substantive revision of the 1982 ANA publication, *Standards of Psychiatric and Mental Health Nursing Practice* (ANA 1982). The specialty standards contained in this publication provide specific measurement criteria for the clinical practice of psychiatric-mental health nursing and are built on the broader general standards of nursing practice as delineated in the ANA *Standards of Clinical Nursing Practice* (ANA 1991b).

This book provides definitions and descriptions of basic and advanced psychiatric-mental health clinical nursing practice. It delineates the scope, functions, and roles of the clinical practice of psychiatric-mental health nurses as well as the diverse settings in which they practice. In addition, it establishes the clinical practice standards for the specialty. This publication is intended for those who deliver, benefit from, and pay for psychiatric-mental health services. It is useful for nurse colleagues and other professionals with an interest in the specialty practice of psychiatric-mental health nursing. Finally, it provides policy makers, insurers, and the public with information about the roles and responsibilities of psychiatric-mental health nurses across the continuum of care.

STATEMENT
on
PSYCHIATRIC-MENTAL HEALTH
CLINICAL NURSING
PRACTICE

CONTEMPORARY ISSUES AND TRENDS

Psychiatric-mental health nursing is both a product of society and a force for social change. As such, the discipline has been evolving from a highly specialized field to a broader, more expansive area of practice that seeks to integrate the biological and the psychosocial domains of the human condition. This evolution is the result of major developments in science, society, health care, and the nursing profession.

Rapid Expansion of Biological Sciences and Technology

The National Institute of Mental Health (NIMH) has proclaimed the 1990s the "Decade of the Brain." This was a response to the phenomenal discoveries in medicine, neuroscience, endocrinology, immunology, and genetics which are providing an understanding of the direct links among brain biochemistry, human functioning, and conditions of health and illness. Also, the creation of sophisticated technology is illuminating the structure and function of the brain. One hundred years after Dr. Sigmund Freud hypothesized about the wonders of the mind, modern scientists have rediscovered the importance of the brain itself as a powerful influence on and complex determinant of human behavior.

With research providing evidence that the most serious mental disorders should be regarded as diseases of the brain, there is a major shift toward the "medicalization" of mental illness (Lowery 1992). The positive side of this shift is that, much as biomedical advances helped conquer many physical illnesses, advances such as magnetic resonance imaging, neurosurgical techniques, psychopharmacology, and genetic therapy hold promise for more effective treatment for those with depression, schizophrenia, anxiety, and other serious mental disorders. These advances foster new hope among mental health providers and consumers that dramatic scientific breakthroughs will produce the means to treat and ultimately prevent many mental illnesses.

Some fear that the pendulum may swing too far in the direction of relying on medical treatments for all psychiatric and mental health problems, to the exclusion of psychotherapeutic interventions. This is unlikely since research to date substantiates the superiority of the combined treatment of psychopharmacology and psychotherapy in severe mental illness to any one treatment by itself.

It is predicted that there will still be a need for psychotherapeutic techniques to help people cope with the psychosocial aspect of acute and chronic mental illness, the effects of stressful lifestyles, dysfunctional interactive patterns, societal problems, aging, serious illness, and their

3

responses to treatment. Also, various approaches such as behavioral, cognitive, dynamic, insight, solution-focused, and system-directed therapies will become more targeted toward specific conditions, and, consequently, will produce even more beneficial and measurable outcomes.

Nurses in psychiatric-mental health practice are in an advantageous position to address the re-integration of physical and psychosocial care for individuals with mental illness (McBride 1990). The emphasis on the connections among brain, spirit, mind, and body is revitalizing psychiatric nursing practice. Psychiatric-mental health nurses are skilled in the specialized use of communication, counseling, and psychotherapeutic techniques. In addition, they incorporate a general practice knowledge stressing the relationship between biological, psychological, social, cultural, spiritual, and environmental factors and health and illness. With continuing education in neuroscience as well as behavioral science, psychiatric-mental health nurses will continue to fine-tune their abilities to assess, diagnose, and treat human responses to a wide spectrum of illnesses.

Demographic Shifts in the Population

A major change in the demographic composition of the population is taking place in America. There is an unprecedented increase in the number of elderly, ethnic minorities, and the economically and educationally disadvantaged. The shift in population fuels tension among different racial, cultural, economic, political, social, educational, and religious groups, profoundly affecting all aspects of society.

There is a concomitant crisis in the mental health of the nation. Not only are more people at risk for and experiencing mental illness related to the pressures of these social conditions, but our understanding of mental illness itself is changing. Some known disorders are evolving into long-term chronic illnesses that drain the energy and resources of families, communities, and the mental health care system. Relatively newly recognized disorders such as Acquired Immune Deficiency Syndrome (AIDS) dementia, post-traumatic stress disorder (PTSD), and chemical dependence in newborns and children, present a challenge to the use of well-established models of treatment and the increasing scarcity of psychiatric care resources (Pothier, Stuart, Puskar, and Babich 1990).

The difficulty in working to solve mental health problems—which frequently are compounded by other problems such as the culture of violence, joblessness, homelessness, teenage pregnancy, illiteracy, and failing physical health—is magnified by the myriad different life experiences, value systems, languages, cultural beliefs, and generational perspectives of those who need mental health services. A further complication is that professional providers often differ significantly from the recipients of their care in terms of these background and experience variables, and hence must be educated more broadly to provide culturally sensitive care.

4

Increasing numbers of psychiatric nurses are working in community-based settings with individuals, families, and communities that are experiencing both the opportunities and challenges which accompany societal shifts and pandemic health care problems. Educational programs are seeking non-traditional clinical placements for psychiatric nursing students and including courses which focus on assessment of strengths and competencies, cultural diversity, healthy aging, short-term therapies, nutrition, and language study to prepare psychiatric nurses for practice with diverse populations.

There is more focus on the developmental issues and mental health needs of men and women, children and adolescents, and the elderly. While women customarily have been a disproportionate part of the patient population in psychiatry, research on female physiology and psychological development suggests that diagnostic and treatment formulations will change to reflect new knowledge.

There is also emphasis on the special needs of rural, homeless, and other underserved populations. This has been encouraged by governmental initiatives and private-sector funding for demonstration projects providing mental health services for these hard-to-reach groups. By focusing on the care of particular age groups (e.g., child, adolescent, and elderly) or populations (e.g., survivors of violence, cocaine-addicted mothers, homeless families, and immigrants), psychiatric nurses are continuing to develop the in-depth knowledge, cultural sensitivity, and therapeutic skills necessary to build new models for care and to design relevant interventions. They are working to establish common ground with those whose needs for psychiatric and mental health care are not being met in the present system. However, there still must be a concerted effort to attract more racial minorities and ethnically diverse individuals to the psychiatric-mental health nursing profession.

Changes in the Delivery of Mental Health Services

Prior to the end of World War II , psychiatric care was delivered in separate facilities, on a long-term basis, and with most of the financing coming from either non-insured private payers or very limited tax-supported programs. This "system" limited individuals' access to care and placed an inordinate emotional and financial burden on their families and communities. Efforts to improve access and develop new models of care in the '60s and '70s eventually failed because of changes in governmental spending priorities, failure of the system to convert to new approaches, and pervasive public attitudes about the stigma surrounding mental illness (Billings 1993).

Since then, a complex sequence of events has changed the nature and delivery of mental health services. These events include the de-institutionalization of tens of thousands of patients from mental hospitals, the subsequent breakdown of the public sector, the skyrocketing inflation of health care costs, the ascendancy of privatization and managed care, and the movement for reform of general health care. The result of these events is a pattern of service delivery which is payer-driven rather than practice-driven in an effort to contain costs.

With a major focus on cost containment, there is evidence that many individuals with serious psychiatric illness remain under-diagnosed and under-treated. Those who are most severely ill are hospitalized in psychiatric intensive-care units where they are treated with psychopharmacologic agents and discharged after a very limited stay. A premium is put on the use of medical intervention. For nurses who provide expert care in these units, the work is complicated by the management of complex behavioral problems of the patients and the pressure to strive for cost containment. Because there is pressure to decrease the patient's length of stay in the hospital, most patients are barely stabilized before they are discharged. Early discharge leads to more acutely ill patients in the community who continue to need expert professional care and intensive case management.

In the future, given the downsizing of specialized psychiatric units and the privatization of outpatient psychiatric care, using a managed-care model, it is predicted that very acutely ill psychiatric patients will be admitted to general hospital units for highly technological diagnostic procedures and aggressive medical treatment, much as patients with serious physical illnesses are admitted to critical-care units now (Lowery 1992). The specialized psychiatric facilities that remain may also become more dependent on this high-tech approach to diagnosis and treatment of mental illness.

Furthermore, the total spectrum of mental health care needs will expand to include health promotion and disease prevention. For example, programs that address healthy parenting, stress management, and learning adaptive coping skills, enhance mental health and may prevent the psychological trauma associated with family violence. Education of young children about the effects of addictive substances may interrupt the cycle of addiction, saving the next generation of children from the effects of psychosocial problems and learning disabilities. There will be an emphasis on the consumer's responsibility and involvement in self-care related to mental health. Nurses will share information so that consumers and families can make informed choices and give input about their care.

Therefore, delivery of mental health care will take place more frequently on an outpatient basis or in community-based settings such as homes, schools, halfway houses—even the streets (Koldjeski 1984). Also, as the brain-mind-body connection becomes better understood, there will be a continuing effort to provide psychosocial care for the physically ill in the community. These trends will reactivate the community mental health movement because its goals dovetail with the federal government's goal to focus on health promotion and disease prevention through the *Healthy People 2000* (HHS 1990) objectives.

These service delivery trends have resulted in the need for psychiatric-mental health nurses to provide primary mental health care. Nurses are alert to opportunities to promote mental health, to detect and intervene in situations with increased stress, developmental crises, and family violence and abuse which often predispose the people involved to mental disorders. Nurses must be able to make rapid comprehensive assessments; use effective problem-solving skills in making complex clinical decisions; act autonomously as well as collaboratively with other professionals; be sensitive to issues such as ethical dilemmas, cultural diversity, and access to mental health care for underserved populations; be comfortable working in decentralized settings; and be sophisticated about the costs and benefits of providing care within fiscal constraints. Psychiatric-mental health nurses have the knowledge, skills, and creativity to adapt their practice to meet the demands of new delivery systems while improving quality mental health care.

There is also a need for psychiatric care to be mainstreamed into the overall health care system. Sweeping changes are forecast for the delivery of all health services in the near future, and reform of the system must include parity for mental health services. It is imperative that those needing mental health services have access and benefits equal to those individuals needing general health care services. In any national health reform legislation there must be equitable coverage based on clinical needs for all mental and physical health care services delivered in managed care systems. Access to care must be enhanced, especially for those who are uninsured and unemployed. (ANA 1991a, Krauss 1993)

Psychiatric-mental health nurses are active as informed individuals and through their professional nursing organizations in the advocacy of increased access, equal treatment and insurance coverage for persons with mental illness and their families. In seeking parity for mental health services, psychiatric nursing organizations have formed partnerships with consumer groups and other professional organizations to educate the public about the similar and unique needs of those with mental health problems.

DESCRIPTION OF PSYCHIATRIC-MENTAL HEALTH NURSING

Psychiatric-mental health nursing is the diagnosis and treatment of human responses to actual or potential mental health problems. Psychiatric-mental health nursing is a specialized area of nursing practice, employing theories of human behavior as its science and purposeful use of self as its art.

Psychiatric-mental health nurses deliver primary mental health care. Primary mental health care is initiated at the first point of contact with the mental health care system. Primary mental health care is defined as the continuous and comprehensive services necessary for promotion of optimal

PSYCHIATRIC-MENTAL HEALTH NURSING'S PHENOMENA OF CONCERN

Actual or potential mental health problems of clients pertaining to:

*the maintenance of optimal health and well-being and the prevention of psychobiologic illness.

*self-care limitations or impaired functioning related to mental and emotional distress.

*deficits in the functioning of significant biological, emotional, and cognitive systems.

*emotional stress or crisis components of illness, pain, and disability.

*self-concept changes, developmental issues, and life process changes.

*problems related to emotions such as anxiety, anger, sadness, loneliness, and grief.

*physical symptoms that occur along with altered psychological functioning.

*alterations in thinking, perceiving, symbolizing, communicating, and decision making.

*difficulties in relating to others.

*behaviors and mental states that indicate the client is a danger to self or others or has a severe disability.

*interpersonal, systemic, sociocultural, spiritual, or environmental circumstances or events which affect the mental and emotional well-being of the individual, family, or community.

*symptom management, side effects/toxicities associated with psychopharmacologic intervention and other aspects of the treatment regimen.

Figure 1.   Psychiatric-Mental Health Nursing's Phenomena of Concern.

mental health, the prevention of mental illness, health maintenance, management of, and/or referral of mental and physical health problems, the diagnosis and treatment of mental disorders and their sequelae, and rehabilitation (Haber and Billings 1993). Because of its scope, psychiatric-mental health nursing is necessarily holistic and considers the needs and strengths of the whole person, the family and the community.

Diagnosis of human responses to actual or potential mental health problems involves the application of theory to human phenomena, through the processes of assessment, diagnosis, planning, intervention or treatment, and evaluation. Theories relevant to psychiatric-mental health nursing are derived from various sources, including those from nursing as well as the biological, cultural, environmental, psychological and sociological sciences. These theories provide a basis for psychiatric-mental health nursing practice.

An assessment, derived from data collection, interview and behavioral observations, provides information upon which a diagnosis is based and, when appropriate, validated with the client. The psychiatric-mental health nurse uses nursing diagnoses and standard classifications of mental disorders such as *The Diagnostic and Statistical Manual of Mental Disorders* of the American Psychiatric Association (American Psychiatric Association 1987) or the *International Classification of Diseases* (World Health Organization 1993) to develop a treatment plan based on assessment data and theoretical premises. The nurse then selects and implements interventions directed toward a client's response to an actual or potential health problem. The nurse periodically evaluates the client outcome and revises the plan of care to achieve optimal results.

PSYCHIATRIC-MENTAL HEALTH NURSING PRACTICE ETHICS

Nursing's respect for the client's dignity, autonomy, cultural beliefs, and privacy is of particular concern in psychiatric-mental health nursing practice. The nurse serves as an advocate for the client and is obliged to demonstrate nonjudgemental and nondiscriminatory attitudes and behaviors that are sensitive to client diversity. Unethical behavior—e.g., violations of informed consent, breaches of confidentiality, undue coercion, and illegal acts—can increase the client's vulnerability demanding special vigilance on the part of the nurse who is responsible to protect the client and to report practices which compromise the public's right to humane and appropriate care. Nurses working with psychiatric-mental health clients are prepared to recognize the special nature of the provider-patient relationship and take steps to assure therapeutic relationships are conducted in a manner that dheres to the mandates stipulated in the *Code for Nurses* (ANA 1980).

SCOPE OF PSYCHIATRIC-MENTAL HEALTH CLINICAL NURSING PRACTICE

The scope of psychiatric-mental health nursing practice is differentiated according to the nurse's level of practice and further delineated by the role of the nurse and the work setting. It is the responsibility of individual nurses to identify their practice parameters within their state nurse practice act, professional code, and professional practice standards, and, according to their own personal competency, to perform particular activities or functions. The nurse's competence is circumscribed by the individual nurse's education, knowledge, experience, and abilities. While psychiatric-mental health nurses are accountable for their own nursing practice, as professionals they have a responsibility to collaborate and to coordinate care with others who may be working with the client and with those whose expertise can enhance the quality of service.

LEVELS OF PSYCHIATRIC-MENTAL HEALTH CLINICAL NURSING PRACTICE

Psychiatric-mental health nurses are registered nurses (RNs) who are educationally prepared in nursing and licensed to practice in their individual states. Registered nurses are qualified for specialty practice at two levels—basic and advanced. These levels are differentiated by educational preparation, professional experience, type of practice, and certification. In addition, these levels can differ based on the nurse's focus on clinical, administrative, educative, and research roles. This book is confined to a statement which addresses the clinical role, scope and standards of practice in the specialty area of psychiatric-mental health nursing.

Basic Level

Psychiatric-Mental Health Registered Nurse. The Psychiatric-Mental Health Nurse is a licensed RN who has a baccalaureate degree in nursing and demonstrated clinical skills, within the specialty, exceeding those of a beginning RN or a novice in the specialty. The designation, Psychiatric-Mental Health Nurse, applies to those nurses who are certified within the specialty and who meet the profession's standards of knowledge and experience. Certification is the formal process that validates the nurse's clinical competence. The letter "C," placed after the R.N. (i.e., R.N., C.), is the initial that designates basic-level certification status.

Many professional nurses who contribute to the practice of psychiatric-mental health nursing and care for mental health clients are either entry level RNs or are novices in the specialty. These nurses practice in conjunction with psychiatric-mental health nurses and are responsible for adhering to the specialty practice standards as designated by the profession.

Advanced Level

Psychiatric-Mental Health Advanced Practice Registered Nurse. The Psychiatric-Mental Health Advanced Practice Registered Nurse (APRN) is a licensed RN who is educationally prepared at the master's level, at a minimum, and is nationally certified as a clinical specialist in psychiatric and mental health nursing. This preparation is distinguished by a depth of knowledge of theory and practice, supervised clinical practice, and competence in advanced clinical nursing skills. The psychiatric-mental health APRN has the ability to apply knowledge, skills, and experience autonomously to complex mental health problems.

The doctorally prepared psychiatric-mental health nurse in advanced practice has both a master's degree in nursing and a doctorate in nursing or a related field. Academic programs in nursing leading to a doctorate follow one of two traditions: 1) advanced development of the clinical nursing role with a research component directed toward the investigation of specific clinical problems (Doctor of Nursing Science-D.N.Sc.); or 2) research and theory development in the science of psychiatric-mental health nursing (Doctor of Philosophy-Ph.D.).

The scope of practice in psychiatric-mental health nursing is expanding as the context of practice, the need for client access to holistic care, and the various scientific and nursing knowledge bases evolve. Many state legislatures and Congress have acknowledged the unique role of advanced practice psychiatric nurses in the delivery of mental health services by passing legislation which makes them eligible for prescriptive authority, admission privileges, and third-party reimbursement.

Historically, the psychiatric-mental health nurse in advanced practice has been called a *clinical nurse specialist* (CNS). The term *advanced practice registered nurse* (inclusive of the terms clinical nurse specialist, nurse anesthetist, nurse midwife, nurse practitioner) has emerged in response to the need for uniform titling within the nursing profession. The appropriate credential for advanced clinical practice in this specialty is that of the Certified Specialist in Psychiatric and Mental Health Nursing (R.N., C.S.). In this book, the psychiatric-mental health advanced practice nurse is referred to as a *certified specialist*.

SUBSPECIALIZATION

Subspecialization in a specific area of practice occurs during master's and doctorate preparation in nursing and/or through continuing professional education. Subspecialization is focused on the development of additional knowledge and skills for providing services to a population. Subspecializations within psychiatric-mental health nursing emerge based on current and anticipated societal needs for specific specialty nursing services. This subspecialization may be categorized according to a developmental period (e.g. child and adolescent, adult, geriatric) (ANA 1985), a specific mental/emotional disorder (e.g. addiction, depression, chronic mental illness), a particular practice focus (e.g. community, group, couple, family, individuals), and/or a specific role or function (e.g. psychiatric consultation-liaison). These categories are not mutually exclusive but provide a matrix within which the parameters of subspecialization are defined.

Some psychiatric-mental health nurses in advanced practice seek certification in subspecialty areas as a means of obtaining recognition in a particular practice focus. At this time, not all subspecialties are coupled with a certification process, nor is subspecialty certification essential for practice. It is graduate preparation, additional training and experience, and the individual nurse's judgment about readiness to work with a particular situation or client population that constitute appropriate practice.

Given this additional preparation, as long as the nurse is certified as a specialist in an area of psychiatric/mental health nursing, that nurse can appropriately practice in a subspecialty area with or without certification in that area. In other words, subspecialty certification in a particular category of psychiatric-mental health nursing does not confine the certified specialist only to the area of subspecialization. For example, nurses certified as specialists in adult psychiatric and mental health nursing appropriately work with children as part of a family approach either in family therapy or adjunctively in the treatment of adult parents. Similarly, certified specialists in child and adolescent psychiatric and mental health nursing see adults (for example, parents) in therapy.

PSYCHIATRIC-MENTAL HEALTH NURSING CLINICAL PRACTICE FUNCTIONS

Basic Level Functions

The psychiatric-mental health nurse works with individuals, families, groups, and communities to assess mental health needs, develop diagnoses, and plan, implement, and evaluate nursing care. Basic level psychiatric-mental health nursing practice is characterized by interventions that promote and foster health, assess dysfunction, assist clients to regain or improve their coping abilities, and prevent further disability. These interventions focus on psychiatric-mental health clients and include health promotion and health maintenance; intake screening and evaluation; case management; provision of a therapeutic environment (i.e., milieu therapy); tracking clients and assisting them with self-care activities; administering and monitoring psychobiological treatment regimens (including prescribed psychopharmacologic agents and their effects); health teaching; crisis intervention and counseling; and outreach activities such as home visits and community action.

Health Promotion and Health Maintenance. As a primary mental health care provider, the psychiatric-mental health nurse emphasizes health promotion and health maintenance reflecting nursing's long-standing concern for individual, family, group, and community well-being. The psychiatric-mental health nurse conducts health assessments, targets at-risk situations, and initiates interventions such as assertiveness training, stress management, parenting classes, and health teaching, in addition to targeting potential complications related to symptoms of mental illness and adverse treatment effects.

Intake Screening and Evaluation. Psychiatric-mental health nurses function at the point of an individual client's entry into the mental health system, performing intake screening and evaluation including physical and psychosocial assessments, rendering diagnostic and dispositional judgments, and facilitating the client's movement into appropriate services. Data collection at the point of contact involves observational and investigative activities which are guided by the nurse's knowledge of human behavior and the principles of the psychiatric interviewing process. The nurse considers biophysical, psychological, social, cultural, economic, and environmental aspects of the client's life situation to gain an understanding of the problem as it has been experienced and to plan the kind of assistance that is indicated. The nurse is responsible for recognizing areas where additional clinical data are needed and referring the client for more specialized testing and evaluation.

Case Management. Case management is a clinical component of a nurse's role in both inpatient and outpatient settings. Nurses who are case managers support the client's highest level of functioning through culturally relevant interventions designed to enhance self-sufficiency and progress toward optimal health. These can include supportive counseling, problem-solving, teaching, medication and status monitoring, comprehensive care planning, and linkage to and identification and coordination of various other health and human services.

Milieu Therapy. In the practice of milieu therapy, the nurse utilizes the human and other resources of institutional and supervised community-based residential or day treatment settings to foster the restoration of individual clients' previous adaptive abilities and their acquisition of new ones. A key idea in milieu therapy is that virtually all aspects of the therapeutic community, comprised of staff and clients, can exert a major influence on behavior, facilitating or impeding the individual's potential for growth and change. On behalf of individual clients, the psychiatric-mental health nurse assesses and develops the therapeutic potential of a given setting by attending to a wide range of factors such as the physical environment, the social structure and interaction processes, and the culture of the setting.

Similarly, the nurse may practice the use of self as a therapeutic resource through interactions at a one-to-one or group level, in structured or informal sessions, and in the physical as well as the psychosocial aspects of care. Formulation and implementation of the nursing care program proceed from individualized assessments of client needs and involve the client and the client's family and significant others to the fullest extent possible.

Self-Care Activities. A major dimension of direct nursing care functions within the therapeutic milieu involves self-care activities of daily living. Examples of nursing care which takes advantage of the learning potential inherent in the daily life cycle are personal hygiene, feeding, recreational activities, and socialization in practical skills of community life such as shopping and using public transportation. By comforting, guiding, and setting limits, the nurse can make use of clients' experiences of daily living to help them move from dependent to more independent modes of behavior.

Psychobiological Interventions. Another dimension of psychiatric-mental health nursing derives from the understanding and application of psychobiological knowledge bases for psychiatric-mental health nursing care. The nurse's distinctive contribution rests in the ability to evaluate holistically and treat client responses to actual and potential health problems. The psychiatric-mental health nurse employs psychobiological interventions which include various emergency procedures and standard nursing measures such as relaxation techniques, nutrition/diet regulation, exercise and rest schedules, and other somatic treatments, including monitoring of the client's responses to psychobiological interventions and the overall treatment program. Psychobiological interventions also include such activities as the interpretation and implementation of prescriptions related to medication, electroconvulsive therapy, and other treatment regimens.

Nurses in a variety of mental health settings plan and implement services to meet clients' needs for a stable emotional and social support system. A frequent component of these support services is the nurse's support and surveillance of the client's pharmacotherapeutic treatment. These services may be provided on an individual or group basis. The aim is to teach clients about their medications and assist them in dealing with practical problems related to side effects and other difficulties encountered in continuing a prescribed medication regimen while maintaining residence in the community setting.

An essential aspect of the client's response is the right to exercise personal choice about participation in proposed treatments. The nurse's responsible use of authority respects the client's freedom to choose among existing alternatives and facilitates awareness of resources available to assist with decision making.

Health Teaching. Another aspect of the psychiatric-mental health nurse's work with individuals, families, and community groups is health teaching

In performing this function, the nurse integrates knowledge of the principles of teaching and learning with knowledge of health and illness. The need for health teaching may relate to biological, pharmacologic, physical, sociocultural, or psychological aspects of the learner's care. Selection of particular formal and informal learning methods depends on identified needs and learning outcomes. Nurses recognize that experiential learning opportunities are particularly important in developing understanding of mental health problems and skills to cope with them. Constructive role modeling by the nurse is an inherent part of the teaching function.

Crisis Intervention. Psychiatric-mental health nurses provide direct crisis intervention services to persons in crisis and serve as members of crisis teams. Crisis intervention is a short-term therapeutic process that focuses on the resolution of an immediate crisis or emergency through the use of available professional personnel, family, and/or environmental resources.

Counseling. In nursing, the aim of counseling is to focus specifically— and for a limited period of time—with a client, family, or group, on a problem representing an immediate difficulty related to health or well-being. The difficulty is investigated using a problem-solving approach, so that the experience may be understood more fully and integrated with other life experiences.

Home Visit. Psychiatric-mental health nurses utilize the home visit as an effective method of responding to the mental health needs of an individual or family. In this context, the term home refers to private residences or substitute dwellings—e.g. prisons, halfway houses, homes for the disabled, nursing homes, foster care residences, or shelters for the homeless. In some instances, the nurse's insight into a mental health problem and the resources available to cope with it depend on the assessment data available in the home setting. The nurse also may select the home visit as the most efficacious means of intervention by helping to stimulate the potential helping responses of family members or other significant persons. Efforts to help the family adapt to the re-entry of the discharged psychiatric patient into the home environment is another example of the nurse's function within the home setting.

Community Action. Psychiatric-mental health nursing involvement includes community action—i.e., concern for sociocultural factors that adversely affect the mental health of population groups and the design of activities that can ameliorate these problems. The psychiatric-mental health nurse who functions in the life of the community itself often may deal with problems that occur at a wide variety of different points on the health/illness continuum. The practices of these community-oriented nurses vary in the emphasis given to consultation and education aimed at enhancing others' mental health capabilities, on the one hand, and direct therapeutic involvement with clients, on the other hand. Involvement with community planning boards, advisory groups, paraprofessionals and other key people is an important means by which nurses can mobilize the community's resources and bring about changes that address the mental health needs of particular population groups.

Advocacy. A particularly important dimension of the clinical role of psychiatric-mental health nurses is that of the advocate and policy influencer/maker. These nurses have a long history of supporting the cause of one of the most neglected constituencies—those with mental illness. However, there is a need for new energy and political activism. Some nurses are influencing policy by assuming leadership positions in government agencies at the local, state, and federal level, and by running for legislative office.

Others are joining in consumer and professional groups' campaigns to demystify mental illness, abolish the stigma so often attached to it, and achieve parity between mental and physical illness health care coverage. To accomplish this, nurses are engaging in public speaking, writing articles for the popular press, and lobbying their congressional representatives on behalf of better mental health and psychiatric care for all Americans. In clinical practice, the nurse-advocate vigilantly protects the rights of clients and speaks for those who, for whatever reason, cannot speak for themselves. Because of nursing's strong commitment to the health, welfare, and safety of the client, the nurse must be aware of any activity which places the rights or well-being of the client in jeopardy and take appropriate action in the client's behalf.

Advanced Level Functions

While all aspects of the role functions of the psychiatric-mental health nurse at the basic level of practice can be performed by the certified specialist, psychiatric-mental health nursing at the advanced level demands expertise in psychotherapy modalities associated with various client systems (individual, couple, group, family, and community). Along with the nursing focus on the full range of activity from mental health promotion to illness rehabilitation, the advanced practice role also involves additional psychobiologic interventions involved in the diagnosis and treatment of mental disorders. These include the prescription of psychoactive medications and the ordering of appropriate diagnostic and laboratory tests, according to state nursing regulations.

The certified specialist is a primary mental health care provider who is prepared to carry out health promotion activities at the macro-system level. In community mental health and primary care settings, the Certified Specialist in Psychiatric-Mental Health Nursing analyzes the health needs of both individuals and populations and designs programs which target at-risk groups and cultural and environmental factors which foster health and prevent mental illness. Typical activities include the development of and participation in programs such as mobile services for the homeless; suicide prevention projects targeted at school children; substance abuse and violence prevention strategies; rural mental health clinics; and other creative programming which is flexibly oriented to community needs.

The certified specialist combines case management functions with population-specific nursing knowledge coupled with research competencies, expertise in supportive psychotherapy, and the ability to work with complex and severe mental health problems. The result is the mobilization of therapeutic resources and the maximization of positive outcomes.

Certified specialists frequently provide clinical supervision to assist others in further developing their clinical practice skills. The certified specialist may also practice consultation-liaison nursing to provide consultation and direct care services in non-psychiatric settings such as general health care centers.

Psychotherapy. Certified specialists who have demonstrated a high level of competence in psychotherapy by acquiring certification credentials are qualified to assume autonomous responsibility for the primary therapist role. Such nurses are accountable for their own practices and are prepared to perform psychotherapy services independent of any other discipline in the full range of delivery settings. The nurse-therapist's educational preparation in both the biological and social sciences gives that therapist a unique ability to differentiate various aspects of the client's functioning and to make appropriate judgments about the need for interventions, referral, or consultation with other specialists.

Psychotherapy refers to all generally accepted methods of therapy, specifically including individual therapy (e.g., play therapy and other expressive therapies, insight therapy, behavioral therapy; brief and long-term therapy, goal or solution-oriented therapy, and cognitive therapy), group therapy, couple/marital therapy, and family therapy. Psychotherapy denotes a formally structured, contractual relationship between the therapist and client(s) for the explicit purpose of effecting change in the client system. This approach attempts to treat mental disorders, alleviate emotional distress, reverse or change maladaptive behavior, and facilitate personal growth and development.

The therapeutic contract with the client is structured in the beginning phase of the therapy relationship. Included in the terms of the contract are such elements as purpose, time, place, fees, the individuals participating, confidentiality, and access to emergency after-hours assistance. To assure quality, the nurse must continually scrutinize the therapy sessions in relation to the content, process, and rationales for therapeutic judgments and actions.

Proficiency in the art and science of psychotherapy is an outgrowth of advanced, specialized educational experience and of efforts to refine psychotherapy skills through practice, continuing education, and the use of competent consultation with other psychotherapists. This consultation minimizes personal inferences on the part of the therapist, and enhances the therapist's competence in the conduct and evaluation of therapy.

The various psychotherapies (individual, family, and group) are distinguished by who receives the care. Even though individual psychotherapy is variable in the theories and techniques employed by different therapists, it does possess some stable, common elements. It is a relationship between two persons who engage in a confidential, and primarily (for adults) verbal, series of interactions, over an identified period of time, with the agreed upon purpose of change on the part of the client. Experienced certified specialists who have developed skills in individual psychotherapy are qualified to teach and provide clinical consultation to other professionals or psychotherapy training programs.

Family and marital (couple) therapy has as its primary focus and goal the improvement of the couple or family system of interaction. The certified specialist acting as a family therapist can use a variety of approaches to enhance the function of the family's patterns of communication and relationship. Family diagnosis, interventions, and outcome evaluations emphasize the observable, interrelated behaviors that characterize the family system. Nurses who acquire specialized preparation in family therapy have the advantage of building on prior nursing education and experience in which family-centered orientations are developed. These nurse family therapists are qualified to offer clinical supervision to other therapists who work with families and to teach family therapy content and methods.

In group psychotherapy, the dynamics of behavior in small groups is purposefully used to foster exploration of adjustment patterns and to discover more effective and realistic behavioral alternatives. In the role of group therapist, the certified specialist utilizes knowledge of behavior at the intrapersonal, interpersonal, and group levels. Experienced certified specialists who have developed skills in group work are qualified to function as teachers and clinical supervisors in group therapy training programs.

Psychobiological Interventions. Psychobiological interventions include a range of therapies from diet/nutrition regulation, hypnosis, and relaxation techniques to the use of pharmacologic agents. The focus of these interventions is to integrate physiological and psychological dimensions of care and to improve the client's psychological well-being and ability to function.

The clinical role of the certified specialist may incorporate the prescribing of pharmacologic agents to promote the client's optimum functioning. In this role, the nurse applies biological, immunological, neurobiological, pharmacological, and physiological knowledge in assessment and planning strategies. The certified specialist who has prescriptive authority functions in accordance with the state practice act and state and federal regulations.

Clinical Supervision/Consultation. Clinical supervision/consultation is an educative and consultative function of the advanced practice clinical role. Through professional preparation and clinical experience the certified specialist is qualified to provide clinical supervision at the request of other mental health providers and provider-trainees. Clinical supervision/consultation is based on many factors, including knowledge of human behavior and symptomatology and an understanding of the variations of human behavior through which pathology is expressed, familiarity with advanced therapeutic techniques, competency in clinical case management through all phases of the therapeutic process, and expertise in the dynamics of the supervisory process itself. Certified specialists who function as clinical supervisors maintain and improve their own competencies by giving direct care to selected clients, thus serving as clinical role models as well as clinical consultants.

Consultation-Liaison. Consultation-liaison nursing is another primary mental-health advanced nursing practice role in psychiatric and non-psychiatric settings. The clinical aspect of this role ranges from mental health promotion to illness rehabilitation. In consultation-liaison activities, the certified specialist focuses on the emotional, spiritual, developmental, cognitive, and behavioral responses of clients who enter the health care system with actual or potential physical dysfunction. The psychiatric consultation-liaison nurse makes psychiatric and psychosocial diagnoses and implements a wide variety of interventions with physically ill or disabled clients and families. These certified specialists also function in the indirect care roles of consultant and educator with nurses and other health care providers who are consultees in a variety of physical care delivery systems. (ANA 1990)

PSYCHIATRIC-MENTAL HEALTH NURSING CLINICAL PRACTICE SETTINGS

There are two principle arrangements for the clinical practice of psychiatric-mental health nursing: organized health care settings and self-employment. Nurses who work within organized settings are paid for their services on a salaried, contractual, or fee-for-service basis. The settings and arrangements for psychiatric-mental health nursing practice vary widely in purpose, type, location, and the auspices under which they are operated.

Consistent with the concepts of the community mental health movement, nurses seek to position themselves on the basis of the client's right of access to needed services and to the fullest possible use of nursing knowledge and skills. As nurses have increased their contributions to a full range of mental health services, they have become more flexibly deployed in a variety of settings with responsibility for providing mental health care to individuals, families, and communities.

Some nurses enter the social environments which are integral parts of people's daily lives—homes, schools, and work sites—to provide mental health services. Community-based psychiatric-mental health nurses are pivotal in providing primary mental health care and preserving the supports which facilitate family and social network functioning. The community-based settings where these nurses practice include, but are not limited to, educational and judicial system programs, home-health agencies, employee assistance programs, mental health clinics, health maintenance organizations, primary care centers, clinics for the homeless, senior centers, emergency and crisis centers, day care shelters for battered women and children, and soup kitchens and shelters for individuals with chronic mental illness. The versatility of the psychiatric-mental health nurse promotes the development of a wide variety of linkages for access to mental health services.

Psychiatric-mental health nurses practice effectively in a range of intermediate- and long-term care settings which exist for treatment and support of those with severe and persistent mental disorders. These include day- and night-care services, residential care facilities, rehabilitation settings, and therapeutic foster care as well as other innovative service delivery programs. Nurses continue to practice in more traditional psychiatric treatment settings such as general hospitals, psychiatric units of community hospitals, centers for detoxification and the treatment of chemical dependence, psychiatric rehabilitation facilities, private inpatient settings, and the publicly funded hospital system. An important focus for the nurse is to assist in the client's transition from the institutional to the community setting.

Self-employed certified specialists offer direct services in solo private practice and group practice settings, or through contracts with employee assistance programs, health maintenance organizations, managed care companies, preferred provider organizations, industry health departments, home-health agencies, or other service delivery arrangements. In these settings, the certified specialist provides primary mental health care to clients in the nurse's caseload. These nurses also may form nurse-owned corporations or organizations which can compete with other provider groups for mental health service contracts with industries or employers.

CONCLUSION

By defining, clarifying, and reviewing the clinical practice of psychiatric-mental health nursing, this statement contributes to the further development of nursing practice and education. It emphasizes the strong influence nurses have on health promotion, illness prevention, and the provision of comprehensive care. By attesting to the significant nursing contributions to mental health care delivery, this document reflects psychiatric-mental health nursing's responsiveness to the needs of the consumer of mental health services.

Standards of Psychiatric-Mental Health Clinical Nursing Practice

INTRODUCTION

This section of the book sets forth standards of professional clinical practice for the specialty of psychiatric-mental health nursing. Standards are authoritative statements in which the nursing profession describes the responsibilities for which nurses are accountable. Consequently, standards reflect the values and priorities of the profession. Standards provide direction for professional nursing practice and a framework for the evaluation of practice. Written in terms of measurable criteria, standards also define the nursing profession's accountability to the public and the client outcomes for which nurses are responsible. Standards are relatively enduring, while the criteria by which they are measured may change to reflect new knowledge and technology in current practice.

Standards of Psychiatric-Mental Health Clinical Nursing Practice describes a competent level of professional nursing care and professional performance common to nurses engaged in psychiatric-mental health nursing practice in any setting. These standards apply to nurses who are qualified by education and experience to practice at either the basic level or the advanced level of psychiatric-mental health nursing. Since some nursing activities are highly dependent on variables such as client situation, clinical setting, and instances of individual judgment, language such as "as appropriate," "when possible," and "as applicable" is used to recognize circumstances where exceptions may occur.

Standards of Psychiatric-Mental Health Clinical Nursing Practice applies to the care that is provided to all clients. *Clients* can include an individual, family, group, or community for whom the nurse is providing formally specified psychiatric-mental health services as sanctioned by state nursing practice acts. This care may be provided in the context of health promotion, disease or injury prevention, health maintenance, or health restoration. The cultural, racial, spiritual/religious, and ethnic heritage of the client must always be respected and taken into account in providing psychiatric-mental health nursing services.

The professional practice of psychiatric-mental health nursing is characterized by the application of relevant theories to explain human behavior and related phenomena and to provide a basis for nursing intervention and evaluation of client-oriented health outcomes. The psychiatric-mental health nurse's critical thinking and selective use of theoretical knowledge and research provides for the comprehensive biopsychosocial assessment and accurate diagnosis of the client's response to actual or potential mental health problems and for analysis of the reciprocal interaction between client and environment.

Theory and research also guide the nurse's analysis of data, choice of interventions, methods of implementation, and evaluation of client outcomes, as well as the application of theory to practice. To sustain and build on theory-based practice, psychiatric-mental health nurses, in their practice settings, must have resource materials in that setting, support for and access to continuing education programs, and a philosophy that is congruent with theory-based nursing actions.

Standards of Clinical Practice in Psychiatric-Mental Health Nursing has two sections. The first includes those standards related to the direct clinical care the patient receives, as demonstrated through the nursing process. ANA calls these "Standards of Care." The second is "Standards of Professional Performance," which describes a competent level of behavior in the professional role.

STANDARDS OF CARE

"Standards of Care" pertain to professional nursing activities that are demonstrated by the nurse through the nursing process. These involve assessment, diagnosis, outcome identification, planning, implementation, and evaluation. The nursing process is the foundation of clinical decision making and encompasses all significant action taken by nurses in providing psychiatric-mental health care to all clients.

Standard I. Assessment

THE PSYCHIATRIC-MENTAL HEALTH NURSE COLLECTS CLIENT HEALTH DATA.

Rationale

The assessment interview—which requires linguistically and culturally effective communication skills, interviewing, behavioral observation, database record review, and comprehensive assessment of the client and relevant systems—enables the psychiatric-mental health nurse to make sound clinical judgments and plan appropriate interventions with the client.

Measurement Criteria

1. The priority of data collection is determined by the client's immediate condition or need.
2. The data may include but are not limited to:
    a. ability to remain safe and not be a danger to oneself and others.
    b. client's central complaint, symptoms, or focus of concern.
    c. physical, developmental, cognitive, mental, and emotional health status.
    d. history of health patterns and illness.
    e. family, social, cultural, and community systems.
    f. daily activities, functional health status, substance use, health habits, and social roles, including work and sexual functioning.
    g. interpersonal relationships, communication skills, and coping patterns.
    h. spiritual or philosophical beliefs and values.
    i. economic, political, legal, and environmental factors affecting health.
    j. significant support systems, both available and underutilized.
    k. health beliefs and practices.
    l. knowledge, satisfaction, and motivation to change, related to health.
    m. strengths and competencies that can be used to promote health.
    n. other contributing factors that influence health.
3. Pertinent data are collected from multiple sources using various assessment techniques and standardized instruments as appropri-

ate. Multiple sources of assessment data can include not only the client, but also family, social network, other health care providers, past and current medical records, and community agencies and systems (with consideration of the client's confidentiality).

4. The client, significant others, and interdisciplinary team members are involved in the assessment process to the extent possible.
5. The client and significant others are informed of their respective roles and responsibilities in the assessment process and data analysis.
6. The assessment process is systematic and ongoing.
7. The data collection is based on clinical judgment to ensure that relevant and necessary data are collected.
8. The database is synthesized, prioritized, and documented in a retrievable form.

Standard II. Diagnosis

THE PSYCHIATRIC-MENTAL HEALTH NURSE ANALYZES THE ASSESSMENT DATA IN DETERMINING DIAGNOSES.

Rationale

The basis for providing psychiatric-mental health nursing care is the recognition and identification of patterns of response to actual or potential psychiatric illnesses and mental health problems.

Measurement Criteria

1. Diagnoses and potential problem statements are derived from assessment data.
2. Interpersonal, systemic, or environmental circumstances—that affect the mental well-being of the individual, family, or community—are identified.
3. The diagnosis is based on an accepted framework which supports the psychiatric-mental health nursing knowledge and judgment used in analyzing the data.
4. Diagnoses conform to accepted classifications systems—such as North American Nursing Diagnosis Association (NANDA) Nursing Diagnosis Classification, *International Classification of Diseases* (WHO 1993), and *The Diagnostic and Statistical Manual of Mental Disorders* (APA 1987) used in the practice setting.
5. Diagnoses and risk factors are validated with the client, significant others, and other heath care providers when appropriate and possible.
6. Diagnoses identify actual or potential psychiatric illness and mental health problems of clients pertaining to:
   a. the maintenance of optimal health and well-being and the prevention of psychobiologic illness.

b. self-care limitations or impaired functioning related to mental and emotional distress.
c. deficits in the functioning of significant biological, emotional, and cognitive systems.
d. emotional stress or crisis components of illness, pain, and disability.
e. self-concept changes, developmental issues, and life process changes.
f. problems related to emotions such as anxiety, aggression, sadness, loneliness, and grief.
g. physical symptoms that occur along with altered psychological functioning.
h. alterations in thinking, perceiving, symbolizing, communicating, and decision making.
i. difficulties in relating to others.
j. behaviors and mental states that indicate the client is a danger to self or others or has a severe disability.
k. interpersonal, systemic, sociocultural, spiritual, or environmental circumstances or events which have an affect on the mental and emotional well-being of the individual, family, or community.
l. symptom management, side effects/toxicities associated with psychopharmacologic intervention and other aspects of the treatment regimen.
7. Diagnoses and clinical impressions are documented in a manner that facilitates the identification of client outcomes and their use in the plan of care and research.

Standard III. Outcome Identification

THE PSYCHIATRIC-MENTAL HEALTH NURSE IDENTIFIES EXPECTED OUTCOMES INDIVIDUALIZED TO THE CLIENT.

Rationale

Within the context of providing nursing care, the ultimate goal is to influence health outcomes and improve the client's health status.

Measurement Criteria

1. Expected outcomes are derived from the diagnoses.
2. Expected outcomes are client-oriented, therapeutically sound, realistic, attainable, and cost-effective.
3. Expected outcomes are documented as measurable goals.
4. Expected outcomes are formulated by the nurse and the client, significant others, and interdisciplinary team members, when possible.
5. Expected outcomes are realistic in relation to the client's present and potential capabilities.

6. Expected outcomes are identified with consideration of the associated benefits and costs.
7. Expected outcomes estimate a time for attainment.
8. Expected outcomes provide direction for continuity of care.
9. Expected outcomes reflect current scientific knowledge in mental health care.
10. Expected outcomes serve as a record of change in the client's health status.

Standard IV. Planning

THE PSYCHIATRIC-MENTAL HEALTH NURSE DEVELOPS A PLAN OF CARE THAT PRESCRIBES INTERVENTIONS TO ATTAIN EXPECTED OUTCOMES.

Rationale

A plan of care is used to guide therapeutic intervention systematically and achieve the expected client outcomes.

Measurement Criteria

1. The plan is individualized, tailored to the client's mental health problems, condition, or needs and it:
   a. identifies priorities of care in relation to expected outcomes.
   b. identifies effective interventions to achieve the outcomes.
   c. specifies interventions that reflect current psychiatric-mental health nursing practice and research.
   d. includes an education program related to the client's health problems, treatment, and self-care activities.
   e. indicates responsibilities of the psychiatric-mental health nurse and the client, and may include responsibilities for inter-disciplinary team members to carry out the plan of care.
   f. gives direction for client-care activities delegated by the psychiatric-mental health nurse to other care providers.
   g. provides for appropriate referral and case management to insure continuity of care.
2. The plan is developed in collaboration with the client, significant others, and interdisciplinary team members, when appropriate.
3. The plan is documented in a manner that allows access to it by team members and modification of the plan as necessary.

Standard V. Implementation

THE PSYCHIATRIC-MENTAL HEALTH NURSE IMPLEMENTS THE INTERVENTIONS IDENTIFIED IN THE PLAN OF CARE.

Rationale

In implementing the plan of care, psychiatric-mental health nurses use a wide range of interventions designed to prevent mental and physical illness, and promote, maintain, and restore mental and physical health. Psychiatric-mental health nurses select interventions according to their level of practice. At the basic level, the nurse may select counseling, milieu therapy, self-care activities, psychobiological interventions, health teaching, case management, health promotion and health maintenance, and a variety of other approaches to meet the mental health needs of clients. In addition to the intervention options available to the basic-level psychiatric-mental health nurse, at the advanced level the certified specialist may provide consultation, engage in psychotherapy, and prescribe pharmacologic agents where permitted by state statutes or regulations.

Measurement Criteria

1. Interventions are selected based on the needs of the client and accepted nursing practice.
2. Interventions are selected according to the psychiatric-mental health nurse's level of practice, education, and certification.
3. Interventions are implemented within the established plan of care.
4. Interventions are performed in a safe, ethical, and appropriate manner.
5. Interventions are documented.

Standard Va. Counseling

THE PSYCHIATRIC-MENTAL HEALTH NURSE USES COUNSELING INTERVENTIONS TO ASSIST CLIENTS IN IMPROVING OR REGAINING THEIR PREVIOUS COPING ABILITIES, FOSTERING MENTAL HEALTH, AND PREVENTING MENTAL ILLNESS AND DISABILITY.

Measurement Criteria

1. Counseling interventions—including communication and interviewing techniques, problem-solving skills, crisis intervention, stress management, relaxation techniques, assertiveness training, conflict resolution, and behavior modification—are documented.
2. Counseling reinforces healthy behaviors and interaction patterns and helps the client modify or discontinue unhealthy ones.
3. Counseling promotes the client's personal and social integration.

Standard Vb. Milieu Therapy

THE PSYCHIATRIC-MENTAL HEALTH NURSE PROVIDES, STRUCTURES, AND MAINTAINS A THERAPEUTIC ENVIRONMENT IN COLLABORATION WITH THE CLIENT AND OTHER HEALTH CARE PROVIDERS.

Measurement Criteria

1. The client is familiarized with the physical environment, the schedule of activities, and the norms and rules that govern behavior and activities of daily living, as applicable.
2. Current knowledge of the effects of the client's environment is used to guide nursing actions.

3. The therapeutic environment is designed utilizing the physical environment, social structures, culture, and other available resources.
4. Communication among clients and staff supports an effective milieu.
5. Specific activities are selected that meet the client's physical and mental health needs.
6. Limits of any kind (e.g., restriction of privileges, restraint, seclusion, timeout) are used in a humane manner, are the least restrictive necessary, and are employed only as long as needed to assure the safety of the client and of others.
7. The client is given information about the need for limits and the conditions necessary for removal of the restriction, as appropriate.
8. The client and significant others are given the opportunity to ask questions and discuss their feelings and concerns about past, current, and projected use of various environments.

Standard Vc. Self-Care Activities

THE PSYCHIATRIC-MENTAL HEALTH NURSE STRUCTURES INTERVENTIONS AROUND THE CLIENT'S ACTIVITIES OF DAILY LIVING TO FOSTER SELF-CARE AND MENTAL AND PHYSICAL WELL-BEING.

Measurement Criteria

1. The self-care interventions assist the client in assuming personal responsibility for activities of daily living.
2. The self-care activities of daily living are appropriate for the client's age, developmental level, gender, sexual orientation, ethnic/social background, and education.
3. Self-care interventions are aimed at maintaining and improving the client's functional status.

Standard Vd. Psychobiological Interventions

THE PSYCHIATRIC-MENTAL HEALTH NURSE USES KNOWLEDGE OF PSYCHOBIOLOGICAL INTERVENTIONS AND APPLIES CLINICAL SKILLS TO RESTORE THE CLIENT'S HEALTH AND PREVENT FURTHER DISABILITY.

Measurement Criteria

1. Current knowledge of psychopharmacology and other psychobiological therapies are used to guide nursing action.
2. Psychopharmacological agents' intended actions, untoward effects, and therapeutic doses are monitored, as are blood levels where appropriate.
3. The client's responses to therapies serve as clinical indications of treatment effectiveness.
4. Nursing interventions are directed toward alleviating untoward effects of psychobiological interventions, when possible.
5. Opportunities are provided for the client and significant others to question, discuss, and explore their feelings about past, current, and projected use of therapies.

6. Nursing observations about the client's response to psychobiological interventions are communicated to other health providers.

Standard Ve. Health Teaching

THE PSYCHIATRIC-MENTAL HEALTH NURSE, THROUGH HEALTH TEACHING, ASSISTS CLIENTS IN ACHIEVING SATISFYING, PRODUCTIVE, AND HEALTHY PATTERNS OF LIVING.

Measurement Criteria

1. Health teaching is based on principles of learning.
2. Health teaching includes information about coping, interpersonal relations, mental health problems, mental disorders, and treatments and their effects on daily living, as well as information pertinent to physical status or developmental needs.
3. The nurse uses health teaching methods appropriate to the client's age, developmental level, gender, ethnic/social background, and education.
4. Constructive feedback and positive rewards reinforce the client's learning.
5. Practice sessions and experiential learning are used as needed.

Standard Vf. Case Management

THE PSYCHIATRIC-MENTAL HEALTH NURSE PROVIDES CASE MANAGEMENT TO COORDINATE COMPREHENSIVE HEALTH SERVICES AND ENSURE CONTINUITY OF CARE.

Measurement Criteria

1. Case management services are based on a comprehensive approach to the client's physical, mental, emotional, and social health problems.
2. Case management services are provided in terms of the client's needs and the accessibility, availability, quality, and cost-effectiveness of care.
3. Health-related services and more specialized care are negotiated as needed—on behalf of the client—with the appropriate agencies and providers.
4. Relationships with agencies and providers are maintained throughout the client's use of the health care services to ensure continuity of care.
5. The client's decisions related to the plan of care and treatment choices are supported, as appropriate.

Standard Vg. Health Promotion and Health Maintenance

THE PSYCHIATRIC-MENTAL HEALTH NURSE EMPLOYS STRATEGIES AND INTERVENTIONS TO PROMOTE AND MAINTAIN MENTAL HEALTH AND PREVENT MENTAL ILLNESS.

Measurement Criteria

1. Health promotion and disease prevention strategies are based on knowledge of health beliefs, practices, and epidemiological principles, along with the social, cultural, and political issues that affect mental health in an identified community.
2. Health promotion and disease prevention interventions are designed for clients identified as at-risk for mental health problems.
3. Consumer participation is encouraged in identifying mental health problems in the community and planning, implementing, and evaluating programs to address those problems.
4. Community resources are identified to assist consumers in using prevention and mental health care services appropriately.

Advanced Practice Interventions Vh-Vj

The following interventions (Vh-Vj) may be performed only by the certified specialist in psychiatric-mental health nursing.

Standard Vh. Psychotherapy

THE CERTIFIED SPECIALIST IN PSYCHIATRIC-MENTAL HEALTH NURSING USES INDIVIDUAL, GROUP, AND FAMILY PSYCHOTHERAPY, CHILD PSYCHOTHERAPY, AND OTHER THERAPEUTIC TREATMENTS TO ASSIST CLIENTS IN FOSTERING MENTAL HEALTH, PREVENTING MENTAL ILLNESS AND DISABILITY, AND IMPROVING OR REGAINING PREVIOUS HEALTH STATUS AND FUNCTIONAL ABILITIES.

Measurement Criteria

1. The therapeutic contract with the client is structured to include:
    a. purpose, goals, and expected outcomes.
    b. time, place, and frequency of therapy.
    c. fees and payment schedule.
    d. participants involved in therapy.
    e. confidentiality.
    f. availability and means of contacting therapist.
    g. responsibilities of both client and therapist.
2. Knowledge of personality theory, growth and development, psychology, psychopathology, social systems, small-group and family dynamics, stress and adaptation, and theories related to selected therapeutic methods is used, based on the client's needs.
3. Therapeutic principles are used to understand and interpret the client's emotions, thoughts, and behaviors.
4. The client is helped to deal constructively with thoughts, emotions, and behaviors.
5. Increasing responsibility and independence are fostered in the client to reinforce healthy behaviors and interactions.

6. Continuity of care is provided in therapist's absence.
7. Nursing care for the client's physical needs is referred to another provider when it is determined that such care provided by the therapist would impair the client/therapist relationship.

Standard Vi. Prescription of Pharmacologic Agents

THE CERTIFIED SPECIALIST USES PRESCRIPTION OF PHARMACOLOGIC AGENTS IN ACCORDANCE WITH THE STATE NURSING PRACTICE ACT, TO TREAT SYMPTOMS OF PSYCHIATRIC ILLNESS AND IMPROVE FUNCTIONAL HEALTH STATUS.

Measurement Criteria

1. Prescriptive authority for pharmacologic agents is used only by those nurses who are qualified by education and experience and in accordance with the state nursing practice act or state and federal regulations.
2. Psychoactive pharmacologic agents are prescribed based on a knowledge of psychopathology, neurobiology, physiology, immunology, expected therapeutic actions, anticipated side effects, and courses of action for unintended or toxic effects.
3. Specific pharmacological agents are prescribed based on clinical indicators of the client's status, including the results of diagnostic and laboratory tests, as appropriate.
4. Information about intended effects, potential side effects of the proposed prescription, and alternative treatments is provided to the client.

Standard Vj. Consultation

THE CERTIFIED SPECIALIST PROVIDES CONSULTATION TO HEALTH CARE PROVIDERS AND OTHERS TO INFLUENCE THE PLANS OF CARE FOR CLIENTS, AND TO ENHANCE THE ABILITIES OF OTHERS TO PROVIDE PSYCHIATRIC AND MENTAL HEALTH CARE AND EFFECT CHANGE IN SYSTEMS.

Measurement Criteria

1. Consultation activities are based on models of consultation, systems principles, communication and interviewing techniques, problem-solving skills, change theories, and other theories as indicated.
2. A working alliance, based on mutual respect and role responsibilities, is established with the consultee.
3. The decision to implement the system change or plan of care remains the responsibility of the consultee.

Standard VI. Evaluation

THE PSYCHIATRIC-MENTAL HEALTH NURSE EVALUATES THE CLIENT'S PROGRESS IN ATTAINING EXPECTED OUTCOMES.

Rationale

Nursing care is a dynamic process involving change in the client's health status over time, giving rise to the need for new data, different diagnoses, and modifications in the plan of care. Therefore, evaluation is a continuous process of appraising the effect of nursing interventions and the treatment regimen on the client's health status and expected health outcomes.

Measurement Criteria

1. Evaluation is systematic and ongoing.
2. The client, significant others, and team members are involved in the evaluation process, as possible, to ascertain the client's level of satisfaction with care and evaluate the cost and benefits associated with the treatment process.
3. The client's responses to interventions are documented.
4. The effectiveness of interventions in relation to outcomes is evaluated.
5. Ongoing assessment data are used to revise diagnoses, outcomes, and the plan of care as needed.
6. Revisions in the diagnoses, outcomes, and the plan of care are documented.
7. The revised plan provides for continuity of care.

STANDARDS OF PROFESSIONAL PERFORMANCE

"Standards of Professional Performance" describe a competent level of behavior in the professional role, including activities related to quality of care, performance appraisal, education, collegiality, ethics, collaboration, research, and resource utilization. All psychiatric-mental health nurses are expected to engage in professional role activities appropriate to their education, position, and practice setting. Therefore, some standards or measurement criteria identify these activities.

While "Standards of Professional Performance" describe the roles of all professional nurses, there are many other responsibilities that are hallmarks of psychiatric-mental health nursing. These nurses should be self-directed and purposeful in seeking necessary knowledge and skills to enhance career goals. Other activities—such as membership in professional organizations, certification in specialty or advanced practice, continuing education, and further academic education—are desirable methods of enhancing the psychiatric-mental health nurse's professionalism.

Standard I. Quality of Care

THE PSYCHIATRIC-MENTAL HEALTH NURSE SYSTEMATICALLY EVALUATES THE QUALITY OF CARE AND EFFECTIVENESS OF PSYCHIATRIC-MENTAL HEALTH NURSING PRACTICE.

Rationale

The dynamic nature of the mental health care environment and the growing body of psychiatric nursing knowledge and research provide both the impetus and the means for the psychiatric-mental health nurse to be competent in clinical practice, to continue to develop professionally, and to improve the quality of client care.

Measurement Criteria

1. The psychiatric-mental health nurse participates in quality-of-care activities as appropriate to the nurse's position, education, and practice environment. Such activities can include:
   a. identification of aspects of care important for quality monitoring— e.g., functional status, symptom management and control, health behaviors and practices, safety, client satisfaction, and quality of life.
   b. identification of indicators used to monitor the effectiveness of psychiatric-mental health nursing care.
   c. collection of data to monitor quality and effectiveness of psychiatric-mental health nursing care.
   d. analysis of quality data to identify opportunities for improving psychiatric-mental health nursing care.
   e. formulation of recommendations to improve psychiatric-mental health nursing practice or client outcomes.
   f. implementation of activities to enhance the quality of psychiatric-mental health nursing practice.
   g. participation on interdisciplinary teams which evaluate clinical practice or mental health services.
   h. development of policies and procedures to improve quality psychiatric-mental health care.
2. The psychiatric-mental health nurse seeks feedback from the client and significant others about their satisfaction with care.
3. The psychiatric-mental health nurse uses the results of quality-of-care activities to initiate changes in psychiatric-mental nursing practice.
4. The psychiatric-mental health nurse uses the results of quality-of-care activities to initiate changes throughout the mental health care delivery system, as appropriate.

Standard II. Performance Appraisal

THE PSYCHIATRIC-MENTAL HEALTH NURSE EVALUATES OWN PSYCHIATRIC-MENTAL HEALTH NURSING PRACTICE IN RELATION TO PROFESSIONAL PRACTICE STANDARDS AND RELEVANT STATUTES AND REGULATIONS.

Rationale

The psychiatric-mental health nurse is accountable to the public for providing competent clinical care and has an inherent responsibility as a professional to evaluate the role and performance of psychiatric-mental health nursing practice according to standards established by the profession and regulatory bodies.

Measurement Criteria

1. The psychiatric-mental health nurse engages in performance appraisal of own clinical practice and role performance with peers or supervisors on a regular basis, identifying areas of strength as well as areas for professional/practice development.
2. The psychiatric-mental health nurse seeks constructive feedback regarding own practice and role performance from peers, professional colleagues, clients, and others.
3. The psychiatric-mental health nurse takes action to achieve goals identified during performance appraisal and peer review, resulting in changes in practice and role performance.
4. The psychiatric-mental health nurse participates in peer review activities when possible.

Standard III. Education

THE PSYCHIATRIC-MENTAL HEALTH NURSE ACQUIRES AND MAINTAINS CURRENT KNOWLEDGE IN NURSING PRACTICE.

Rationale

The rapid expansion of knowledge pertaining to basic and behavioral sciences, technology, information systems, and research requires a commitment to learning throughout the psychiatric-mental health nurse's professional career. Formal education, continuing education, certification, and experiential learning are some of the means the psychiatric-mental health nurse uses to enhance nursing expertise and advance the profession.

Measurement Criteria

1. The psychiatric-mental health nurse participates in educational activities to improve clinical knowledge, enhance role performance, and increase knowledge of professional issues.
2. The psychiatric-mental health nurse seeks experiences and independent learning activities to maintain and develop clinical skills.
3. The psychiatric-mental health nurse seeks additional knowledge and skills appropriate to the practice setting by participating in educational programs and activities, conferences, workshops, and interdisciplinary professional meetings.
4. The psychiatric-mental health nurse documents own educational activities.
5. The psychiatric-mental health nurse seeks certification when eligible.

Standard IV. Collegiality

THE PSYCHIATRIC-MENTAL HEALTH NURSE CONTRIBUTES TO THE PRO-
FESSIONAL DEVELOPMENT OF PEERS, COLLEAGUES, AND OTHERS.

Rationale

The psychiatric-mental health nurse is responsible for sharing knowledge, research, and clinical information with colleagues, through formal and informal teaching methods, to enhance professional growth.

Measurement Criteria

1. The psychiatric-mental health nurse uses opportunities in practice to exchange knowledge, skills, and clinical observations with colleagues and others.
2. The psychiatric-mental health nurse assists others in identifying teaching/learning needs related to clinical care, role performance, and professional development.
3. The psychiatric-mental health nurse provides peers with constructive feedback regarding their practices.
4. The psychiatric-mental health nurse contributes to an environment that is conducive to clinical education of nursing students, as appropriate.

Standard V. Ethics

THE PSYCHIATRIC-MENTAL HEALTH NURSE'S DECISIONS AND ACTIONS ON BEHALF OF CLIENTS ARE DETERMINED IN AN ETHICAL MANNER.

Rationale

The public's trust and its right to humane psychiatric-mental health care are upheld by professional nursing practice. The foundation of psychiatric-mental health nursing practice is the development of a therapeutic relationship with the client. The psychiatric-mental health nurse engages in therapeutic interactions and relationships which promote and support the healing process. Boundaries need to be established to safeguard the client's well-being and to prevent the development of intimate or sexual relationships.

Measurement Criteria

1. The psychiatric-mental health nurse's practice is guided by the *Code for Nurses*.
2. The psychiatric-mental health nurse maintains a therapeutic and professional relationship with clients at all times
3. The psychiatric-mental health nurse maintains client confidentiality and appropriate professional boundaries.
4. The psychiatric-mental health nurse functions as a client advocate.
5. The psychiatric-mental health nurse delivers care in a nonjudgmental and nondiscriminatory manner sensitive to client diversity.

6. The psychiatric-mental health nurse identifies ethical dilemmas that occur within the practice environment and seeks available resources to help formulate ethical decisions.
7. The psychiatric-mental health nurse reports abuse of clients' rights, and incompetent, unethical, and illegal practices.
8. The psychiatric-mental health nurse participates in obtaining the client's informed consent for procedures, treatments, and research, as appropriate.
9. The psychiatric-mental health nurse discusses with the client the delineation of roles and the parameters of the relationship.
10. The psychiatric-mental health nurse carefully manages self-disclosure.
11. The psychiatric-mental health nurse does not promote or engage in initimate or sexual relationships with current clients.
12. The psychiatric-mental health nurse avoids sexual relationships with clients or former clients and recognizes that to engage in such a relationship is unusual and an exception to accepted practice.

Standard VI. Collaboration

THE PSYCHIATRIC-MENTAL HEALTH NURSE COLLABORATES WITH THE CLIENT, SIGNIFICANT OTHERS, AND HEALTH CARE PROVIDERS IN PROVIDING CARE.

Rationale

Psychiatric-mental health nursing practice requires a coordinated, ongoing interaction between consumers and providers to deliver comprehensive services to the client and the community. Through the collaborative process, different abilities of health care providers are used to solve problems, communicate, and plan, implement, and evaluate mental health services.

Measurement Criteria

1. The psychiatric-mental health nurse collaborates with the client, significant others, and health care providers in the formulation of overall goals, plans, and decisions related to client care and the delivery of mental health services.
2. The psychiatric-mental health nurse consults with other health care providers on client care, as appropriate.
3. The psychiatric-mental health nurse makes referrals—including provisions for continuity of care—as needed.
4. The psychiatric-mental health nurse collaborates with other disciplines in teaching, consultation, management, and research activities as opportunities arise.

Standard VII. Research

THE PSYCHIATRIC-MENTAL HEALTH NURSE CONTRIBUTES TO NURSING AND MENTAL HEALTH THROUGH THE USE OF RESEARCH.

Rationale

Nurses in psychiatric-mental health nursing are responsible for contributing to the further development of the field of mental health by participating in research. At the basic level of practice, the psychiatric-mental health nurse uses research findings to improve clinical care and identifies clinical problems for research study. At the advanced level, the psychiatric-mental health nurse engages and/or collaborates with others in the research process to discover, examine, and test knowledge, theories, and creative approaches to practice.

Measurement Criteria

1. The psychiatric-mental health nurse uses interventions substantiated by research as appropriate to the nurse's position, education, and practice environment.
2. The psychiatric-mental health nurse participates in research as appropriate to the nurse's position, education, and practice environment. Such activities can include:
   a. identification of clinical problems suitable for psychiatric-mental health nursing research.
   b. participation in data collection.
   c. participation in unit, organization, or community research committees or programs.
   d. sharing research activities with others.
   e. conducting research and disseminating findings.
   f. critiquing research for application to practice.
   g. using research findings in the development of policies, procedures, and guidelines for client care.
   h. consulting with research experts and colleagues as necessary.
3. The psychiatric-mental health nurse participates in human-subject protection activities as appropriate and is particularly cognizant of the needs of the vulnerable group served.

Standard VIII. Resource Utilization

THE PSYCHIATRIC-MENTAL HEALTH NURSE CONSIDERS FACTORS RELATED TO SAFETY, EFFECTIVENESS, AND COST IN PLANNING AND DELIVERING CLIENT CARE.

Rationale

The client is entitled to psychiatric-mental health care which is safe, effective, and affordable. As the cost of health care increases, treatment decisions must be made in such a way as to maximize resources and maintain quality of care. The psychiatric-mental health nurse seeks to provide cost-effective quality care by using the most appropriate resources and delegating care to the most appropriate, qualified health care provider.

Measurement Criteria

1. The psychiatric-mental health nurse analyzes factors related to safety, effectiveness, and cost when two or more practice options would result in the same expected client outcome.
2. The psychiatric-mental health nurse discusses benefits and cost of treatment options with the client, significant others, and other providers, as appropriate.
3. The psychiatric-mental health nurse assists the client and significant others in identifying and securing appropriate services available to address health-related needs.
4. The psychiatric-mental health nurse assigns tasks or delegates care based on the needs of the client and the knowledge and skills of the selected provider.
5. The psychiatric-mental health nurse participates in ongoing resource utilization review.

REFERENCES

American Nurses Association. 1967. *Statement on psychiatric and mental health nursing practice.* Kansas City, MO: the Author.

———. 1976. *Statement on psychiatric and mental health nursing practice.* Kansas City, MO: the Author.

———. 1980. *Code for nurses.* Kansas City, MO: the Author.

———. 1982. *Standards of psychiatric and mental health nursing practice.* Kansas City, MO: the Author.

———. 1985. *Standards of child and adolescent psychiatric and mental-health nursing practice.* Kansas City, MO: the Author.

———. 1990. *Standards of psychiatric consultation-liaison nursing practice.* Kansas City, MO: the Author.

———. 1991a. *Nursing's agenda for health care reform.* Kansas City, MO: the Author.

———. 1991b. *Standards of clinical nursing practice.* Kansas City, MO: the Author.

American Psychiatric Association. 1987. *Diagnostic and statistical manual of mental disorders (third edition, revised).* Washington, DC: the Author.

Billings, C. V. 1993, February. The possible dream of mental health reform. *The American Nurse* 25 (2), 5.

Haber, J., and Billings, C. 1993. Primary mental health care: A vision for the future of psychiatric-mental health nursing. *ANA Council Perspectives* 2 (2), 1.

Koldjeski, D. 1984. *Community mental health nursing: Directions in theory & practice.* New York: John Wiley & Sons.

Krauss, J. 1993. Health care reform: Essential mental health services. Washington, DC: American Nurses Publishing.

Lowery, B.J. 1992. Psychiatric nursing in the 1990s and beyond. *Journal of Psychosocial Nursing* 30, 7–13.

McBride, A.B. 1990. Psychiatric nursing in the 1990n. *Archives of Psychiatric Nursing* IV (1), 21–28.

Pollner, I.C., Stuart, G.W., Puskar, K., and Babich, K. 1990. Dilemmas and directions for psychiatric nursing in the 1990s. *Archives of Psychiatric Nursing* IV (5), 284–91.

U.S. Department of Health and Human Services, U.S. Public Health Service. 1990. *Healthy people 2000: National health promotion and disease prevention.* Washington, DC: U.S. Government Printing Office.

World Health Organization. 1993. *International classification of diseases* (10th edition). Geneva: the Author.

Worley, N.K., Drago, L., and Hadley, T. 1990. Improving the physical health-mental health interface for the chronically mentally ill: Could nurse case managers make a difference? *Archives of Psychiatric Nursing* IV (2), 108–11.

GLOSSARY

Activities of daily living

Self-care activities—such as eating, personal hygiene, dressing, recreational activities, and socialization—that are performed daily by healthy individuals as part of independent living. During periods of illness, individuals may not be able to perform some or all of these self-care activities.

Allied/ancillary personnel

Non-nurse health care workers, such as nursing assistants and licensed practical nurses (LPNs).

Assessment

The systematic process of collecting relevant client data for the purpose of determining actual or potential health problems and functional status. Methods used to obtain data include interviews, observations, physical examinations, review of records, and collaboration with colleagues.

Brief therapy

Treatment that focuses on the resolution of a specific problem or behavior in a limited number of sessions.

Case management

An intervention in which health care is integrated, coordinated, and advocated for individuals, families, and groups who require services. The aim of case management is to decrease fragmentation and insure access to appropriate, individualized, and cost-effective care. As a case manager, the nurse has the authority and accountability required to negotiate with multiple providers and obtain diverse services.

Certification

The formal process by which clinical competence is validated in a specialty area of practice.

Certified Specialist in psychiatric-mental health nursing (RN, CS)

A psychiatric-mental health clinical nurse specialist who is nationally certified and qualified for autonomous advanced practice.

Client/client system

The individual, family, group, or community for whom the nurse is providing formally specified services.

Clinical supervision/consultation

The process in which one mental health professional seeks assistance from another to discuss therapeutic issues or to identify or clarify a concern or problem and to consider alternatives available for problem resolution.

Counseling	A specific, time-limited interaction of a nurse with a client, family, or group experiencing immediate or ongoing difficulties related to their health or well-being. The difficulty is investigated using a problem-solving approach for the purpose of understanding the experience and integrating it with other life experiences.
Crisis intervention	A short-term therapeutic process that focuses on the rapid resolution of an immediate crisis or emergency using available personnel, family, and/or environmental resources.
Critical Path	A standard written plan and timetable for care that identifies routine treatments, activities, medications, expected length of stay, and discharge planning.
Diagnostic and Statistical Manual of Mental Disorders	Published by the American Psychiatric Association, the manual provides a listing of official diagnostic classifications for mental disorders. Each disorder is classified on one of five Axes—I and II include all clinical syndromes and personality disorders, III contains physical disorders, and IV and V provide information about psychosocial stressors and adaptive functioning.
Family and marital therapy	Approaches used to enhance the family's or couple's relationship and patterns of communication. Diagnoses, interventions, and outcomes emphasize the observable, interrelated behaviors that characterize the family or couple system.
Functional status	Level of the client's ability to perform independently activities related to self-care, social relations, occupational functioning, and use of leisure time.
Holistic treatment	Provision of comprehensive care that identifies physical, emotional, social, economic, and spiritual needs as they relate to the individual's response to illness and to the ability to perform activities of daily living.
Illness trajectory	The course of the illness or chronic condition, which depends on the individual, the interventions utilized, and unpredictable events that occur during the illness' course.
Interventions	Nursing activities that promote and foster health, assess dysfunction, assist clients to regain or improve their coping abilities, and

prevent further disabilities—e.g., conducting intake screening and evaluation; delivering case management services; maintaining a therapeutic environment (i.e., milieu therapy); tracking and assisting with self-care activities; administering and monitoring treatment regimens and their effects, including prescribed psychopharmacologic agents; providing health education; intervening and counseling during a crisis; and providing outreach activities.

Managed care

Spans a broad continuum of entities, from the simple requirement of prior authorization for a service in an indemnity health insurance plan, to the assumption of all legal, financial, and organizational risks for the provision of a set of comprehensive benefits to a defined population. Also, the management of health care clinical services supplied by groups of providers with the aims of cost-effectiveness, quality, and accessibility.

Mental disorder/illness

A disturbance in thoughts or mood that causes maladaptive behavior, inability to cope with normal stresses, and/or impaired functioning. Etiology may include genetic, physical, chemical, biological, psychological, or sociocultural factors.

Mental health

State of well-being in which individuals function well in society and are generally satisfied with their lives.

Milieu therapy/therapeutic environment

A type of psychotherapy using the total environment to provide a therapeutic community. The emphasis is on developing the therapeutic potential of the setting by developing the physical surroundings, structured activities, a stable social structure, and cultural setting to promote interactions and personal growth.

Non-deferrable care

Treatment that cannot be postponed.

Nurse practice act

State statutes that define the legal limits of practice for registered nurses.

Nursing diagnosis classification

A name, taxonomy label, or summarizing group of words that conveys a nursing assessment conclusion regarding actual or potential health problems of the client. Identifying a nursing diagnosis involves a clinical judgment that the problem being addressed is one that nurses have the legal authority to treat.

Nursing practice standards	Authoritative statements that describe a level of care or performance, common to the profession of nursing, by which the quality of nursing practice can be judged. They include activities related to assessment, diagnosis, outcome identification, planning, implementation, evaluation, quality of care, performance appraisal, education, collegiality, ethics, collaboration, research, and resource utilization.
Nursing process	A systematic and interactive problem-solving approach that includes individualized patient/client assessment, planning, implementation/intervention, and evaluation.
Outcome	The client's goal, or the result of interventions, that includes the degree of wellness and the continued need for care, medication, support, counseling, education.
Pathophysiology	The body's biological and physical processes which result in observable signs and symptoms.
Phenomena of concern	Actual or potential mental problems that are of concern to psychiatric-mental health nurses.
Prescriptive authority	The statutory/regulatory authority to prescribe drugs and devices as a component of a profession's scope of practice.
Primary mental health care	A mode of service delivery that is initiated at the first point of contact with the mental health care system. It involves the continuous and comprehensive mental health services necessary for promotion of optimal mental health, prevention of mental illness, and intervention, health maintenance, and rehabilitation.
Professional code	Statement of ethical guidelines for nursing behavior that serves as a framework for decision making.
Psychiatric-mental health nursing	A specialized area of nursing practice that employs theories of human behavior as its science and the purposeful use of "self" as its art. It is the diagnosis and treatment of human responses to actual or potential mental disorders and their long-term effects. Interventions include the continuous and comprehensive primary mental health care services necessary for the promotion of optimal mental health, the prevention of mental illness, rehabilitation from mental disorders, and health maintenance.

Psychiatric-mental health registered nurse	A baccalaureate-prepared registered nurse who demonstrates clinical skills exceeding those of a beginning registered nurse or novice in the specialty and who is employed in the specialized practice of psychiatric-mental health nursing (see "Psychiatric-mental health nursing"). This designation is for those who are nationally certified within the specialty. In this basic practice level, the nurse can function in clinical, administrative, consultative, educative, research, and advocacy roles.
Psychopathology	The mind's biological and physical processes which result in observable signs and symptoms of mental disorder.
Psychopharmacologic agents	Medications used to treat mental disorders.
Psychosocial domain	The range of diagnoses and treatments that are related to mental health, social status, and functional ability.
Psychotherapy	A formally structured, contractual relationship between the therapist and client(s) for the purpose of effecting change in the client system. Approaches include all generally accepted and respected methods of therapy, including individual therapy (play and other expressive therapies, insight therapy, behavioral therapy, cognitive therapy, and brief goal- or solution-oriented therapy), group therapy, couple/marital therapy, and family therapy.
Registered nurse (RN)	An individual educationally prepared in nursing and licensed by the state board of nursing to practice nursing in that state. Registered nurses may qualify for specialty practice at two levels—basic and advanced. These levels are differentiated by educational preparation, professional experience, type of practice, and certification.
Scope of practice	A range of nursing functions that are differentiated according to level of practice, role of the nurse, and work setting. The parameters are determined by each state's nursing practice act, professional code of ethics, and nursing practice standards, as well as each individual's personal competency to perform particular activities or functions.
Psychobiological interventions	Interventions—e.g., relaxation techniques, hypnosis, nutrition and dietary regulations, exercise, rest schedules, and pharmacologic

	agents—used to improve well-being and functioning.
Therapeutic community	The physical environment, clients, staff, and policies of the therapeutic facility, which have an influence on individual functioning in the activities of daily living.
Therapeutic process	Use of the nurse/client relationship and the nursing process to promote and maintain a client's adaptive coping responses.
Therapeutic use of self	Individualized interventions in which the nurse uses theory and experiential knowledge along with self-awareness in assisting clients to explore their impact on others. The goal of therapeutic use of self is the facilitation of behavior change in the client.